BIOLOGICAL TRANSCENDENCE AND THE TAO

Carlos Andromeda
Biological Transcendence and the TAO

All rights reserved
Copyright © 2023 by Carlos Andromeda

Published by BooxAi
ISBN: 978-965-578-385-8

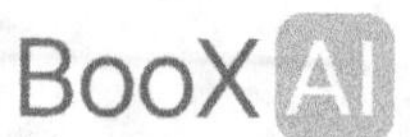

BIOLOGICAL TRANSCENDENCE AND THE TAO

AN EXPOSÉ ON THE POTENTIAL TO ALLEVIATE DISEASE AND AGEING AND THE CONSIDERATIONS OF AGE-OLD WISDOM

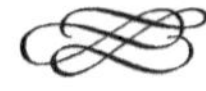

CARLOS ANDROMEDA

Written in tandem with ChatGPT
Prompted and Edited by Carlos Andromeda on
August 7th, 2023

Delve into this exploration of Taoist philosophy
and its interplay with modern medicine as we
contemplate transcending our biological
boundaries via the collective voice of humanity.

CONTENTS

INTRODUCTION

Medicine's Brave New World

As dawn breaks on the 21st century, humanity stands on the brink of what could be termed the "Golden Era" of medicine. Advances in science and technology, which once existed solely in speculative fiction, are rapidly materializing into tangible realities. Our understanding of the human body, combined with technological prowess, is redefining the boundaries of what's possible in healthcare, offering a beacon of hope to countless individuals across the globe.

Yet, with this exhilarating wave of progress comes an undercurrent of profound questions and dilemmas. Can we, in our quest for health and longevity, also ensure that the spirit and ethics of medicine remain intact? How do we navigate this intricate dance between innovation and introspection, ensuring that our advances serve not just the few but the many?

This exposé aims to chart the landscape of modern medicine, diving deep into its most promising avenues—from the regenerative wonders of stem cells to the analytical might of artificial intelligence. But beyond the sheer mechanics and marvels, it also seeks to probe the soul of our collective medical endeavour. We will grapple with the ethical quandaries posed by these advancements, recognizing that the path to medical utopia is fraught with challenges that require scientific acumen and moral wisdom.

Join us on this journey as we explore a world where the age-old dreams of alleviating disease and extending life come face to face with the complex realities of ethics, equity, and humanity's timeless values. Welcome to the brave new world of medicine.

In this dawn where science gleams so bright,
A Golden Era rises, full of might.
Yet as we tread paths once unknown,
Ethics and spirit must be our cornerstone.

Between marvels and soul, we tread a line,
Balancing wonder with the divine.
For in our quest to heal and thrive,
It's the heart of medicine we must keep alive.

As dreams meet reality's vast expanse,
Together, in this intricate dance,
We seek a world both just and true,
With timeless values guiding all we do.

CHAPTER 1: THE GENETICS OF AGEING

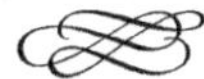

In a labyrinth of cells, DNA, and proteins, the key to human longevity and vitality might just be hiding in plain sight. To grasp the mechanisms of ageing, we must delve into the world of genetics, the science of our very essence.

The Telomere Tale: A Journey Beyond Biological Boundaries

Within the intricate microscopic universe of every human cell, there lies a fascinating story woven around DNA—the building blocks of life. These DNA strands, neatly packed into structures called chromosomes, bear a close resemblance to a tightly coiled book of life's secrets. And, at the very tips of these chromosomes, we find structures termed 'telomeres,' our biological bookends. Analogous to the aglets on our shoelaces, telomeres are crucial in ensuring our DNA remains protected and doesn't deteriorate.

Every time our cells undergo division, a natural and essential process for growth and repair, these telomeres experience a slight reduction in length. It's akin to the wear and tear a book endures with frequent use. Over time, with multiple cell divisions, these telomeres become critically short. The result? The protective covers can no longer shield our precious DNA, instigating a chain reaction of cellular ageing and, ultimately, cell death.

In the vibrant decade of the 1980s, a groundbreaking discovery shook the scientific community: an enzyme named 'telomerase.' This enzyme bore the remarkable ability to replenish and extend these shrinking telomeres. The implications were profound. Could the manipulation of telomerase represent the elusive fountain of youth, promising an extended lifespan and a reversal of cellular ageing? Early experiments heightened this excitement. Cells introduced to telomerase not only saw rejuvenated telomeres but also exhibited traits reminiscent of their younger, more vibrant counterparts.

Several potential paths emerged:

1. **Cellular Rejuvenation Therapies:** By strategically introducing telomerase into ageing cells, researchers envisaged therapies that could renew tissue vitality, potentially offering treatments for age-related diseases or even organ rejuvenation.

2. **Lifespan Extension:** If telomere shortening is intrinsically linked to ageing, then maintaining telomere length could potentially prolong the

human lifespan, offering us more years of healthy, productive life.

3. **Stem Cell Potency:** Telomerase could play a role in enhancing the potency of stem cells, which are cells with the ability to become various cell types. This would be pivotal in regenerative medicine, aiding in repairing damaged tissues or organs.

However, as with all potent tools, wielding telomerase demands caution. A shadow loomed on the horizon: the menace of cancer. Cancer cells, notorious for their uncontrolled growth, often have heightened telomerase activity, enabling them to divide indefinitely. Thus, the puzzle became intricate. Could we utilize telomerase to counteract ageing without inadvertently promoting cancer?

The telomere tale is more than just a chapter in the book of biological understanding. It's a testament to humanity's undying quest to transcend natural limitations. As researchers continue to unravel this narrative, they tread the delicate balance between the promise of extended youth and the inherent responsibilities such knowledge commands. The journey ahead is filled with potential and caution as we seek to harness the full spectrum of telomerase's power in our pursuit of a healthier, longer life.

DNA Damage, Repair, and the Quest for Biological Mastery:

The intricate helix of our DNA, the source code of life, is under constant assault. From the moment we are born, a myriad of external and internal agents threaten its integrity. Environmental factors, such as the relentless bombardment of UV radiation from the sun or exposure to harmful chemicals, contribute to this wear and tear. Additionally, every time our cells divide and copy their DNA—a process that happens billions of times in our lifetime—there's a potential for tiny copying errors akin to typos in a replicated manuscript.

Luckily, nature has endowed our cells with a set of sophisticated tools: DNA repair mechanisms. Picture these as diligent editors, constantly scanning and correcting the typos to maintain the integrity of the original manuscript. These mechanisms work tirelessly to recognize damaged or mismatched DNA segments and fix them, ensuring that our genetic information remains, for the most part, unchanged.

However, time is a formidable adversary. As the years pass, our cellular editors begin to lose their keenness. Their efficiency in spotting and rectifying errors diminishes, leading to a buildup of these genetic "typos." The consequences of this accumulation are multifaceted. Superficially, it can manifest as the visible signs of ageing—wrinkles, age spots, and the loss of skin elasticity. On a more concerning note, unchecked DNA damage can lead to serious health challenges, including the uncontrolled cell growth we recognize as cancer.

So, how do we counteract this inevitable decline?

Research is fervently exploring the depths of our DNA repair mechanisms. A notable avenue of investigation is the role of specific proteins known to facilitate DNA repair. For instance, proteins like PARP1 and BRCA play crucial roles in detecting and repairing DNA strand breaks. By understanding these proteins better, scientists are developing drugs that can either enhance their natural functions or mimic their actions. Some of these drugs have been tested in animal models with intriguing results, such as increased resistance to DNA-damageing agents and, in some cases, extended healthy lifespans.

Another promising path is gene therapy. By introducing or altering genetic material within a person's cells, we might be able to bolster the natural repair processes or even introduce novel ones. Though in its infancy, advancements in tools like CRISPR-Cas9 offer hope that we could directly edit genes responsible for DNA repair, enhancing our natural defences against age-related diseases.

The horizon of DNA repair research is expansive and promising. As we advance our understanding and harness these tools, the dream of transcending our current biological limitations and achieving not just longer, but healthier lives, inches closer to reality.

In essence deep, where our secrets keep,
A world of potential, vast and profound,
DNA threads weave tales, and intricacies abound.
Chapter 1 was a dance, through a realm so small,
Revealing wonders of genes, and challenges that enthrall.

Telomeres, like bookends, guard our story's close,
Hints of age reversed, in their structure they pose.
With each fleeting moment, as they lessen their hold,
Promises of vitality, in their strands unfold.
Yet, amidst this promise, a caution does loom,
Nature's balance stands firm, as cancer might bloom.

Our DNA, a fortress, faces siege day and night,
From errors within, and external blights.
But in tales of frailty, nature's strength shines so bright,
Cellular menders of wounds, in the quiet moonlight.
Time's march may weaken these valiant shields,
But therein lies a call, to untapped fields.

Proteins may bolster, CRISPR may renew,
Boundaries of biology, we aim to eschew.
Yet our quest isn't merely to add to life's days,

But to enrich every moment, in countless ways.

At this genetic brink, we gaze and reflect,
The fabric of our future, with genes intersect.
With understanding and care, we'll etch our new
fate,
Where age's mere digits, and vibrant health won't
abate.

CHAPTER 2: BATTLING THE BIG KILLERS

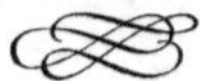

In the ceaseless journey towards a longer and healthier life, modern medicine confronts adversaries that have long claimed countless lives. These formidable foes—cancer, neurodegenerative diseases, heart disease, and diabetes—are intricate in nature, but the battle against them is progressing with tenacity and innovation.

Cancer: The Emperor of All Maladies

Cancer, often referred to as the "Emperor of All Maladies," is a malady that confounds both the medical community and those affected. Its reputation as a formidable foe stems from its inherent nature: it's essentially our own body turning against itself. Picture your cells as diligent workers, each performing their tasks in harmony. But sometimes, a few go astray, multiplying rampantly and not heeding the body's rules. This anarchic behaviour forms the root of cancer. The fight against this malady is an intricate dance, especially since we're battling against a part of ourselves.

Yet, as ominous as this may sound to the average reader, there's hope on the horizon. Medical breakthroughs have opened new doors, providing innovative solutions to this age-old problem. Let's break it down:

Challenges:

1. **Unpredictability**: Every individual's cancer is unique, making it difficult to predict its behaviour and progression. Two people with the same type of cancer might respond differently to the same treatment.

2. **Resistance**: Over time, some cancers can become resistant to treatments, which means that they learn to fend off the therapeutic interventions we use, making them harder to combat.

3. **Side Effects**: Current cancer treatments, like chemotherapy, often have severe side effects because they can't distinguish between healthy cells and cancer cells, leading to collateral damage.

Innovative Solutions:

1. **CAR T-cell Therapies**: Think of this as training an elite squad within your body's defence forces. Your own immune cells, particularly the T-cells, are reprogrammed in a laboratory to recognize the traitorous cancer cells. Once reintroduced into your body, these "special forces" T-cells act like guided missiles, specifically seeking out and destroying the cancerous invaders. This targeted approach minimizes damage to healthy cells, reducing side effects.

2. **CRISPR Technology**: To put it simply, imagine if we had a microscopic pair of scissors that could snip out the bad parts of our genetic code. That's essentially what CRISPR-Cas9 does. It's a revolutionary tool that lets scientists target and "edit" specific genes. By cutting out or fixing the faulty genetic instructions that lead to cancer, we nip the problem in the bud. This means potentially preventing cancer before it even starts.

These advances symbolize our evolving understanding of cancer. While challenges persist, there's a renewed sense of optimism buoyed by the promise of these cutting-edge treatments. The battle against the "Emperor of All Maladies" is fierce, but with continued research and innovation, we march forward, hopeful for a world with fewer cancer-related sorrows.

Neurodegenerative Diseases: Battling the Silent Thieves

Neurodegenerative diseases, like Alzheimer's and Parkinson's, insidiously infiltrate the lives of millions globally. Termed as 'silent thieves,' they gradually strip individuals of cherished memories, precise motor skills, and, ultimately, the essence of their identity. The sheer intricacy of the human brain, with its vast network of synapses and neurotransmitters, renders these ailments particularly formidable to tackle. However, the intersection of science, technology, and holistic health approaches is painting a more optimistic future.

Decoding the Culprits:

- **Amyloid-beta Plaques in Alzheimer's:** One of the defining characteristics of Alzheimer's disease is the buildup of amyloid-beta plaques. Think of these as clutter accumulating in the brain's pathways, disrupting the flow of messages and causing memory lapses.

- **Dopamine Deterioration in Parkinson's:** Parkinson's primarily stems from the decline of dopamine-producing cells. Dopamine is akin to a messenger in the brain, crucial for smooth and coordinated muscle movements. Its depletion leads to the tremors and rigidity synonymous with Parkinson's.

Emerging Medical Frontiers:

- **Targeted Drug Therapies:** Several groundbreaking drugs are under development and testing. Some aim to clear the brain of these detrimental amyloid-beta plaques, acting like a cleanup crew to ensure smoother communication between brain cells. Others focus on Parkinson's, aiming to either supplement dopamine levels or shield the brain's dopamine-producing cells from damage.

- **Gene Therapies:** Leverageing the advancements in genetic engineering, some researchers are venturing into gene therapies. By modifying or replacing faulty genes, they hope to either halt or reverse the progression of these neurodegenerative conditions.

Harnessing Preventative Strategies:

- **Lifestyle Interventions:** A potent arsenal against these diseases lies in our daily routines.

Diets rich in antioxidants, like the Mediterranean diet, have been linked to reduced risks of neurodegenerative diseases. Physical activity, particularly aerobic exercises, enhances brain health by improving blood flow and neural connectivity.

- **Cognitive Training**: Engageing in mentally stimulating activities—be it puzzles, reading, or learning a new skill—fortifies the brain's resilience. By constantly challenging the brain, we can potentially delay the onset or progression of cognitive decline.

- **Community and Social Engagement**: Building and maintaining strong social connections have profound effects on mental well-being. Regular interactions and community engagements act as buffers, reducing stress and enhancing cognitive reserves.

Looking Ahead: Transcending Biological Limitations:

As we delve deeper into the intricacies of the brain, a multifaceted approach emerges. It's not just about developing potent drugs but also about fostering environments and lifestyles conducive to mental longevity. Collaborative efforts—uniting neuroscientists, geneticists, healthcare professionals, and even urban planners and educators—can pave the way for a world where neurodegenerative diseases are not an inevitable part of ageing but anomalies that can be effectively combated.

Heart Disease and Diabetes: Threads of Lifestyle and Genetics

In the tapestry of modern health challenges, heart disease, and diabetes stand out as particularly pronounced threads, often weaving together in a pattern that underscores the impact of contemporary lifestyle choices. These conditions, rising like twin spectres, are largely propelled by the sedentary routines and dietary habits that characterize today's fast-paced world.

The Underlying Dynamics:

- **Interlinked Pathways:** Heart disease and diabetes frequently share a stage, not merely as co-existing conditions but as cause and consequence. For instance, diabetes, by virtue of its impact on blood sugar levels, increases the risk of cardiovascular ailments, including heart attacks and strokes.

- **Dietary Domino Effect:** The omnipresence of processed foods, high in sugars and unhealthy fats, sets off a domino effect. Excessive consumption can lead to obesity, a significant risk factor for both heart disease and diabetes.

The Medical Vanguard:

- **Cutting-Edge Medications:** The pharmaceutical arena is buzzing with innovations. PCSK9 inhibitors, hailed as game-changers, are revolutionizing cholesterol management, substantially mitigating the risk of heart-related events. Meanwhile, the diabetic landscape is being reshaped by drugs like SGLT2 inhibitors, which not only effectively regulate blood sugar but also come with the added advantage of cardiovascular protection.

- **Harnessing the Power of Genetics:** The quest for precision medicine is in full swing. By decoding an individual's genetic blueprint, healthcare is moving towards treatments that are tailored, predicting how one might respond to certain medications, and offering proactive interventions even before diseases manifest.

The Proactive Pathway:

- **Global Health Crusades:** The adage, "Prevention is better than cure," has spurred worldwide campaigns. These initiatives, often supported by health organizations and governments, emphasize the significance of a balanced diet, abundant in fruits, vegetables, and whole grains, and the incorporation of physical activity into daily life.

- **Timely Interventions:** Regular health screenings are being championed more than ever. Detecting potential risk factors or early signs of disease allows for timely interventions, drastically improving outcomes and reducing healthcare burdens.

- **Personalized Health Plans:** With the amalgamation of technology and healthcare, there's a burgeoning trend of personalized health plans. These plans, often facilitated by wearables and apps, offer dietary recommendations, fitness regimes, and even stress-relief techniques, all calibrated to an individual's specific needs.

Forging the Future:

As we navigate this era, marred by the prevalence of heart disease and diabetes, the fusion of global awareness campaigns, medical breakthroughs, and the power of personalized care offers a beacon of hope. By embracing both proactive and reactive measures, there's a promising trajectory toward not just managing, but actively reducing the incidence of these modern-day epidemics.

In the chapter's close, where challenges impose,
Reflect, we must, on both highs and lows.
Each page tells of battles, both fierce and profound,
Yet in every line, our spirit is found.

Diseases loom large, casting shadows so deep,
But humanity's light, its promises keep.
In the face of darkness, our brilliance does gleam,
Uniting and fighting, we chase the same dream.

From the grip of cancer to the heart's silent plea,
Neuro woes and sugar highs, our battles aren't
free.
Yet, these aren't just tales of medicinal might,
They're sagas of souls, in the toughest of fights.

Communities, families, hands clasped tight,
Researchers in labs, seeking answers by night.
For every challenge, a stride we make,
With each discovery, a new dawn we wake.

The path may be steep; the ascent might be rough,
But our steps are firm, our resolve is tough.
A world we envision, free of disease's chain,
Where thriving, not just surviving, is the ultimate
gain.

With optimism in action, hope rooted in truth,
We march forward, from elder to youth.
In this grand tale, we each have a part,
For a healthier world, let the journey start.

CHAPTER 3: REGENERATIVE MEDICINE AND STEM CELLS

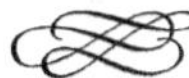

In our pursuit of health and vitality, we arrive at a frontier that seems almost unbelievable in its promises: the realm of regenerative medicine. Here, the dream is not just to treat or manage diseases, but to replace, regenerate, and repair damaged tissues and organs. Central to this dream are stem cells, nature's master craftsmen, capable of becoming nearly any cell type in the human body.

The Stem Cell Symphony: A Dance of Potential and Promise

Imagine an orchestra, where each instrument has its role, its unique sound, and its potential to contribute to the overall melody. Stem cells are much like these instruments, possessing unparalleled versatility and offering an array of therapeutic possibilities in the realm of regenerative medicine. Their intrinsic ability to both self-renew and differentiate sets them apart, making them instrumental in the body's continuous performance of growth, repair, and maintenance.

Types of Stem Cells: Tuning the Instruments of Regeneration

1. **Embryonic Stem Cells (ESCs):** Often considered the "maestros" of the stem cell world, these cells are derived from embryos at a very early developmental stage. Their pluripotent nature means they can evolve into virtually any cell type in the human body. This incredible versatility holds tremendous potential for regenerative therapies, from repairing damaged heart tissue to restoring lost neurons in neurodegenerative conditions. However, their use often stirs ethical debates, given that obtaining them involves the destruction of embryos.

2. **Adult Stem Cells (or Somatic Stem Cells):** Think of these as seasoned musicians, specialized yet adaptable. Located in various tissues throughout the body, such as bone marrow, brain, and liver, their primary role is akin to a repair crew, fixing and maintaining the very tissues they reside in. While their potential is vast, it's more limited compared to ESCs. For instance, a stem cell from the liver might only differentiate into liver cells. Nonetheless, research is ongoing to unlock their full therapeutic capacity, with successes like bone marrow transplants already benefiting countless patients.

3. **Induced Pluripotent Stem Cells (iPSCs):** A groundbreaking innovation akin to giving an old instrument a new tune. Scientists discovered a way to revert mature cells, like skin or blood cells, back

to a pluripotent state similar to embryonic stem cells. This means they can then differentiate into numerous cell types. The beauty of iPSCs lies in their derivation; they can be obtained from the patient themselves, potentially sidestepping issues like tissue rejection. Moreover, their creation does not involve embryos, navigating around the ethical concerns associated with ESCs.

Harmonizing Potential with Practicality:

While the potential of stem cells is undeniable, translating this potential into viable treatments requires meticulous research, rigorous testing, and a profound understanding of each stem cell type's intricacies. Challenges like ensuring the controlled differentiation of stem cells and mitigating potential tumour formation risk must be addressed.

However, the horizon is bright. With each passing day, the symphony of stem cells resonates louder, heralding an era where damaged tissues and organs might be repaired not by artificial implants but by the body's own cells, orchestrated to perfection.

Applications in Modern Medicine:

Organ Repair and Replacement: Pioneering the Next Era of Transplant Medicine with Stem Cells
The Dire Need for Donor Organs:
Every year, thousands find themselves on a transplant waiting list, with the clock ticking away as they hope for a match. The scarcity of donor organs is a pressing concern, often making the difference between life and death for many. This shortage, exacerbated by various factors such as an ageing population, increased incidence of organ failures, and limited organ donors, underlines the urgency for alternative solutions.
Stem Cells: The Building Blocks of Life:
Stem cells, often termed nature's blank slate, possess the unique ability to differentiate into a myriad of cell types. This intrinsic property has

catapulted them to the forefront of regenerative medicine, with researchers exploring their potential in creating lab-grown organs. The approach largely involves directing stem cells to differentiate into specific organ cells and then using them to form organ structures.

From Scaffolds to Functional Organs:

A significant advancement in this domain is the use of "scaffolds" or structural frameworks, which can be derived from decellularized organs. By placing stem cells onto these scaffolds, scientists can guide the cells to grow in a specific shape and pattern mimicking natural organs. Over time, with the right nutrients and growth factors, these cells mature, leading to the development of a functional organ.

Benefits of Stem Cell-Derived Organs:

1. **Eliminating Rejection:** As these organs can be cultivated using a patient's cells, it promises a genetic match, drastically reducing the likelihood of organ rejection post-transplantation.

2. **On-Demand Availability:** This technology could potentially shorten, or even eliminate, waiting lists, offering timely transplants and saving numerous lives.

3. **Ethical Advantages:** Bypassing the need for human donors addresses several ethical quandaries associated with organ transplantation, particularly concerns surrounding informed consent and organ trafficking.

Challenges Ahead:

Despite the promising horizons, creating fully functional organs in the lab is an intricate endeavour. Challenges include ensuring complete vascularization (blood vessel formation) within the organ, achieving integration with the recipient's body systems post-transplantation, and scaling up the production process to meet global demands.

The Future Beckons:

The vision of a world where organ shortages are a thing of the past is tantalizingly within reach. As research progresses, stem cell-derived organs might soon become a mainstay in transplant medicine, heralding a new era of hope and healing for patients around the globe.

Tissue Repair: Stem Cells as the Pioneers of Regenerative Healing

The promise of regenerative medicine lies in its potential to restore the structure and function of damaged tissues, offering hope to countless individuals who suffer from debilitating conditions. Stem cells, with their remarkable ability to transform into various cell types, sit at the forefront of this therapeutic revolution, showing promise in a myriad of applications.

Understanding Tissue Damage and Degeneration:

Tissues, whether from injury or disease, often undergo damage that the body struggles to repair. Traditional treatments might alleviate symptoms but may not address the root cause, leaving the underlying damage untreated.

The Role of Stem Cells in Tissue Repair:

Stem cells are the body's raw materials, cells from which other cells with specialized functions are generated. When deployed in regenerative medicine:

1. **Source and Extraction:** Stem cells can be sourced from various places, including bone marrow, adipose tissue, or even the patient's own skin. Their adaptability makes them prime candidates for repairing damaged tissues.

2. **Directed Differentiation:** In controlled environments, stem cells can be coaxed into differentiating into specific cell types needed for repair, such as nerve cells for spinal cord injuries or cardiac cells for heart repair.

3. **Transplantation:** Once the cells are ready, they are introduced to the damaged site, where they integrate with existing tissues and facilitate repair.

Applications in Specific Conditions:

- **Spinal Cord Injuries:** One of the most challenging medical conditions, spinal cord injuries often result in paralysis. Stem cells offer the possibility of regenerating damaged nerve pathways, potentially restoring mobility and sensation. Preliminary trials have shown promising results, with some patients regaining function in previously paralyzed areas.

- **Degenerative Eye Diseases:** Conditions like age-related macular degeneration or retinitis pigmentosa lead to progressive vision loss. Stem cell therapies aim to replace damaged retinal cells, restoring or even enhancing vision. Recent studies have highlighted the potential of stem cells to halt degeneration and, in some cases, improve visual acuity.

- Heart Damage Post-Heart Attacks: After a heart attack, scar tissue often forms, impairing cardiac function. Injecting stem cells into the damaged heart muscle has shown potential in reducing scar tissue and promoting the growth of new blood vessels. This approach aims not only to repair the heart tissue but also to improve the overall functioning of the heart.

Disease Modelling and Drug Testing: Pioneering New Frontiers with iPSCs

The world of modern medicine stands at the cusp of a paradigm shift, thanks in large part to the innovations driven by induced pluripotent stem cells (iPSCs). As a cornerstone of regenerative medicine, iPSCs not only offer therapeutic potential but have transformed the way scientists approach disease modelling and drug testing.

iPSCs are a type of stem cell derived from adult cells that have been genetically reprogrammed back into an embryonic-like pluripotent state. This means they possess the ability to transform into any cell type in the body, mirroring the capability of embryonic stem cells without the associated ethical concerns.

The Revolution in Disease Modelling

Diseases, particularly those of a genetic or degenerative nature, can be challenging to study within the human body due to their complexity. iPSCs offer a unique solution:

-   **Patient-Specific Disease Models:** By reprogramming cells from patients with specific diseases, scientists can develop iPSC-derived cellular models that carry the same genetic makeup as the patient. This allows for the study of the disease's progression in a controlled environment.

- **Understanding Disease Mechanisms:** As these iPSC-derived cells manifest disease characteristics, researchers can observe cellular changes and interactions in real-time. This offers unparalleled insights into disease onset, progression, and underlying cellular malfunctions.

Revolutionizing Drug Testing and Development

Historically, drug development has been a long, expensive, and sometimes inefficient process. Animal models don't always accurately replicate human disease conditions, and clinical trials come with inherent risks. iPSCs are changing this narrative:

- **High-Throughput Drug Screening:** With iPSC-derived disease models, researchers can quickly test thousands of potential drugs to gauge their efficacy. This accelerates the initial stages of drug discovery, potentially bringing effective treatments to the market faster.

-   **Minimizing Clinical Trial Risks:** Before advancing to human trials, potential drugs can be tested on iPSC-derived tissues, offering a more accurate prediction of how they might behave in the human body. This not only reduces potential risks to trial participants but also lowers the chances of late-stage drug failures.

- **Tailored Therapies:** By using patient-specific iPSC models, it's possible to foresee how individual patients might respond to certain treatments. This paves the way for personalized medicine, ensuring patients receive the most effective treatment for their unique genetic makeup.

Ethical and Practical Challenges: Navigating the Complex Landscape of Stem Cell Research

Stem cell research stands at the forefront of modern medicine, offering potential treatments for a myriad of diseases and conditions that were once deemed incurable. However, with these new frontiers come complex challenges, both ethical and practical, that society, researchers, and policy-makers must grapple with.

Dilemmas of Ethical Origins:

- **Embryonic Stem Cells:** The primary ethical controversy in stem cell research centers on the use of embryonic stem cells. These cells are derived from embryos, raising debates about the moral status of the embryo and when life is considered to begin. Many argue that extracting stem cells from an embryo—effectively destroying it in the process—violates the sanctity of life, while others advocate for the potential medical breakthroughs that these cells can offer.

- **Source Consent:** Even when embryos are donated for research purposes, concerns arise about the informed consent process. Ensuring that donors fully understand the implications and potential uses of their donation is vital to ethical research practices.

Tumorigenic Concerns and Safety Issues:

- **Uncontrolled Growth:** One of the remarkable traits of stem cells is their ability to proliferate and differentiate into various cell types. However, if not controlled properly, there's a risk that these cells could grow uncontrollably, leading to tumours. This tumorigenic potential is a significant safety concern, especially for therapies aiming to introduce stem cells into patients.

- **Quality and Purity of Cells:** For stem cell therapies to be safe, the cells used must be of high quality and free from contaminants. Ensuring this purity, especially when scaling up production for broader clinical use, poses a practical challenge.

Translational Challenges: From Bench to Bedside:

- **Replicating Lab Success:** A treatment that works effectively in a controlled lab environment doesn't always translate to the same success in a real-world clinical setting. Factors such as the patient's overall health, the presence of other diseases, and genetic variations can all influence treatment outcomes.

- **Regulatory Hurdles:** Stem cell therapies must undergo rigorous testing and scrutiny before they can be approved for widespread use. Navigating the complex regulatory landscape, which seeks to ensure patient safety, can be a lengthy and re-source-intensive process.

- **Cost Implications:** Developing, testing, and producing stem cell treatments can be incredibly expensive. Addressing how to make these potential treatments affordable and accessible to those in need remains a significant challenge, especially in healthcare systems with limited resources.

In conclusion, while the promise of stem cell research looms large on the medical horizon, the journey to harness its full potential is fraught with complexities. Addressing these ethical and prac-tical challenges is not just the responsibility of re-searchers but also of society at large. Through informed discourse, rigorous safety protocols, and mindful policy-making, the true potential of stem cell therapies can be realized, bringing hope to millions globally.

In the realm where complexity reigns supreme,
Regenerative wonders awake from a dream.
Stem cells, the maestros, lead the grand play,
Repairing, restoring, and lighting the way.

Yet every frontier, brilliant and new,
Holds challenges deep, and questions accrue.
For while there's potential, vast and untapped,

There are ethical paths, yet to be mapped.

The balance is delicate, precise in its need,
Between rapid advancement and caution to heed.
Researchers and policymakers, hand in hand,
Must tread with care on this promising land.

With respect for life, in all of its forms,
Against raging storms, we'll set new norms.
Responsibility and rigour, our guiding light,
In this era of medicine, taking its flight.

A dawn, resplendent, on the horizon gleams,
Stem cell promises more than just dreams.
With thoughtful navigation, side by side,
Humanity stands on a hopeful tide.

CHAPTER 4: TECHNOLOGY AND MEDICINE FUSION

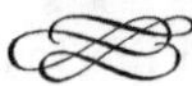

The digital revolution, encapsulating every facet of modern existence, has not left the realm of healthcare untouched. Instead, it's opened up a universe of possibilities, where the fusion of technology and medicine heralds a paradigm shift in how we diagnose, treat, and even anticipate illnesses.

Nanomedicine: Small Scale, Huge Impact

Nanomedicine, the frontier where science meets the microscopic, is poised to revolutionize healthcare. As we delve deeper into the world of the tiny, we discover powerful ways to address medical challenges, making treatments more efficient, safer, and tailored than ever before.

The World of the Tiny:

Nanotechnology and **nanomedicine** are remarkable because they allow scientists to manipulate matter at the atomic or molecular scale, which is roughly 1 to 100 nanometers. To give perspective, a single human hair is about 80,000-100,000 nanometers wide!

Example: **Quantum Dots**, nano-sized semiconductor particles, are being explored for their ability to detect diseases at a very early stage. Their unique property to emit different colours when exposed to light makes them ideal for medical imageing, allowing for earlier and more precise detection of anomalies.

Targeted Drug Delivery:

The brilliance of nanomedicine shines brightly in targeted drug delivery. By using nanoparticles, drugs can be directed precisely where they're needed, minimizing collateral damage to healthy cells.

Example: **Liposomes**, spherical vesicles with at least one lipid bilayer, have been successfully used to deliver chemotherapy drugs directly to cancer cells. Traditional chemotherapy can harm both cancerous and healthy cells, leading to a plethora of side effects. However, with liposome technology, the drugs specifically target cancer cells, sparing the healthy ones and thereby reducing side effects.

Another exciting development is **magnetic nanoparticles**. These can be directed to a specific location using external magnetic fields, making it possible to target drug delivery or heat cancer cells directly without affecting surrounding healthy tissue.

Paths Forward:

1. **Interdisciplinary Collaboration:** The true potential of nanomedicine can be unlocked when

experts from various fields, such as biology, chemistry, physics, and engineering, collaborate. This will accelerate innovation and ensure safety protocols are maintained.

2. **Ethical Considerations:** As with any groundbreaking technology, ethical implications must be addressed. The potential for misuse in areas like human enhancement or bio-weaponry should be guarded against stringent international regulations.

3. **Clinical Trials:** Rigorous testing is paramount. While nanomedicine offers significant benefits, its long-term effects on human health and the environment must be thoroughly understood before widespread application.

4. **Public Awareness and Education:** Educating the public about the potential and challenges of nanomedicine will foster trust and promote its positive applications.

In essence, while the domain of nanomedicine is minuscule in scale, its potential to redefine the boundaries of medical science is colossal. With careful and collaborative steps forward, it promises a healthier, more precise future for all.

Artificial Intelligence and Predictive Healthcare

The integration of Artificial Intelligence (AI) into the healthcare realm has been nothing short of transformative. AI's ability to process vast amounts of data, make predictions, and learn over time offers the promise of a healthcare system that's more efficient, personalized, and proactive. However, like any tool, its true value lies in its judicious and ethical use.

Learning to Heal:

Machine learning (ML), a potent arm of AI, excels in discerning patterns from colossal datasets – a trait invaluable in the healthcare context.

Example: **Radiology and Imageing** have benefited immensely from AI. Tools equipped with ML algorithms can detect subtle abnormalities in X-rays, MRIs, or CT scans that might be missed by the human eye. For instance, Google's DeepMind has developed an AI that can spot eye diseases in scans, predicting the onset of conditions that could lead to blindness.

Another noteworthy application is **epidemiology**. AI models can analyze global health data, weather patterns, and travel trends to predict disease outbreaks, such as influenza or even novel viruses, enabling authorities to take preemptive actions.

Personalized Treatments:

Personalization is at the heart of modern medicine. By harnessing the analytical prowess of AI, treatments can be tailored to fit the unique genetic and lifestyle profile of each patient.

Example: **Genomic Medicine** uses AI to sift through an individual's entire genetic code to identify mutations or anomalies linked to diseases. By understanding these genetic markers, doctors can prescribe treatments or medications that are most likely to be effective for that specific individual.

Moreover, AI-powered wearables and apps can provide real-time health insights, from monitoring heart rates to sleep patterns, allowing individuals to make informed lifestyle choices based on their unique health metrics.

Challenges and Considerations:

While AI is poised to reshape healthcare, it's crucial to be cognizant of the challenges that come with it.

1. **Data Privacy:** With AI processing sensitive health data, there's a pressing need to ensure that this information remains confidential and protected from potential breaches or misuse.

2. **Algorithmic Bias:** AI models are only as good as the data they're trained on. If the training data is skewed or not diverse, the AI can develop biases, leading to misdiagnoses or ineffective treatments for certain populations.

3. **Dependence vs. Expertise:** Relying too heavily on AI might diminish the diagnostic and treatment skills of medical professionals. It's essential to strike a balance, using AI as a supplementary tool rather than a replacement.

4. **Ethical Dilemmas:** The potential to predict diseases or conditions could lead to ethical challenges, such as determining who should have access to predictive information or how it might affect insurance policies.

In conclusion, AI's integration into healthcare offers a tantalizing glimpse into a future where diagnoses are swift, treatments are personalized, and preventative measures are data-driven. Yet, as we stride towards this future, it's imperative to tread with caution, ensuring that the technology is used ethically, equitably, and judiciously.

Biological Transcendence: Wearable and Implantable Tech

The Evolving Nature of Human Biology: In the age of technology, the boundary between human biology and machinery is increasingly blurring. Wearable and implantable devices stand at the forefront of this revolution, symbolizing a future where humans may not just be enhanced by technology but integrated with it.

The Pulse on Your Wrist: The wrist, once a simple appendage for accessories, now functions as a nexus of health information. Modern wearables, such as smartwatches, are constantly evolving, with capabilities that extend beyond monitoring heart rates and sleep patterns. They can now measure blood oxygen levels, detect irregular heart rhythms, and even monitor hydration or stress levels. This avalanche of real-time data not only keeps users informed but can alert them and their healthcare providers to potential issues, shifting the paradigm from treating illnesses to preventing them.

Data-Driven Holistic Wellness: As users get immediate feedback on various health metrics, they're empowered to make lifestyle adjustments in real-time. Over a period, this can lead to more informed choices regarding diet, exercise, and mental health, facilitating a holistic approach to wellness where technology and biology converge.

Beyond Wearables – The Promise of Integration: The horizon of biological transcendence is vast, and wearables are just the beginning. The realm of implantables offers a deeper level of integration. Pioneering research is delving into devices that can be embedded within the body, serving functions such as continuous monitoring of chronic conditions, auto-regulating insulin for diabetics, or even devices that interface with the nervous system to aid in movement or sensory functions. These devices, designed to react in real-time to the body's needs, promise a future where medicine becomes as intrinsic to our biology as any organ.

The Philosophical Implications: As we stand on the precipice of such a transformative era, we must ponder the deeper implications of our journey toward biological transcendence. What does it mean for our identity as humans? How do we ensure the ethical use of such technology? The fusion of biology and tech promises a brighter, healthier future, but it also demands introspection and responsible navigation.

Future Horizons: Telemedicine and the Transformation of Healthcare Accessibility

Reimagining Healthcare Access: Telemedicine has laid the foundation for a future where healthcare transcends borders, both geographical and socioeconomic. Imagine a world where the best doctors aren't limited to elite urban hospitals but are accessible to a shepherd in the mountains or a farmer in a remote village.

Virtual Health Pods: Consider the introduction of "Virtual Health Pods" in public places. These pods, equipped with AI-driven diagnostic tools, could allow patients to step in, undergo a series of tests, and then consult a specialist from anywhere in the world. It would be like having a mini-hospital at every corner, democratizing access to quality healthcare.

Augmented Reality (AR) Assisted Consultations:
With advancements in AR, doctors could potentially "see" patients in a 3D space, allowing for a
more in-depth examination. For instance, a phys-
iotherapist could guide a patient's rehabilitation
exercises by superimposing correct postural align-
ments over the patient's AR display.

AI-powered Predictive Care: Integrating AI with
telemedicine could enable predictive care. Based
on continuous monitoring and data collection, AI
could anticipate health issues before they manifest,
alerting both patient and doctor. This not only aids
in early detection but reshapes the very essence of
medical interventions, focusing more on prevention than cure.

Digital Health Companions: Imagine a personal
AI health companion, available 24/7, equipped to
provide instant medical advice, schedule doctor
appointments, or even offer mental health support.
Such companions could revolutionize daily healthcare, making it personalized, immediate, and om-
nipresent.

Global Medical Collaboration: Telemedicine
platforms could also allow for seamless collaboration among specialists from around the globe, ensuring that patients receive the benefit of multi-
disciplinary expertise, no matter where they are.

Building a Resilient Future: While the COVID-19 pandemic underlined the immediate need for telemedicine, its potential is vast and lasting. As technology continues to advance, the vision for the future of telemedicine is one of global collaboration, accessibility, and proactive care, heralding a new era where distances in healthcare are reduced to mere clicks.

In digital realms where health and code entwine,
A story unfolds, both complex and fine.
From nanoscale wonders to AI's vast might,
Medicine and tech dance in radiant light.

Nanomedicine's whispers, faint but profound,
Seek cures in the places where giants are found.
Tiny warriors armed with purpose and care,
Navigate our veins, healing despair.

While AI, with its vast analytical gaze,
Deciphers' health riddles, guiding our days.
Predictive in power, proactive in quest,
It crafts tailored care, giving only the best.

Upon our very skin, wearables lie,
Syncing with pulses under the sky.
While deeper still, tech integrates within,
A harmonious fusion, where new tales begin.

Telemedicine, with arms that stretch wide,
Brings care to all corners, erasing the divide.
A world where no distance can hamper the care,
Hope reaches all hearts; light fills the air.

Yet as we tread forward, dreams in our sight,
Caution and ethics must guide our flight.
For the dance of tech and medicine's song,
Must respect and uphold, and right any wrong.

In this tale of progress, of humanity's quest,
The fusion of tech and health stands as the best.
In hope, innovation, and care interlaced,
A brighter tomorrow, together, we've embraced.

CHAPTER 5: ETHICAL CONUNDRUMS IN THE MODERN MEDICAL ERA

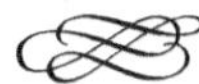

As science and technology propel medicine into unprecedented terrains, a crucial dimension emerges that requires our collective attention: ethics. The possibilities of regenerative medicine, genetic editing, and AI interventions introduce moral dilemmas that challenge the very fabric of our values, societal norms, and philosophical beliefs.

Genetic Engineering: Playing God or Necessary Progress?

The field of genetic engineering is rapidly advancing, pushing the boundaries of science and ethical considerations. At the core of this debate lies the question: Are we playing God, or are we paving the way for a new era of medical and societal progress?

Designer Babies: The rise of technologies like CRISPR has made the once-unthinkable possibility of editing the genes of unborn babies an imminent reality. On the one hand, this holds immense promise: parents could potentially eliminate the risk of debilitating genetic diseases from their child's DNA, ensuring a healthier life ahead. Imagine a world where disorders like Tay-Sachs or Cystic Fibrosis are things of the past.

However, this technology's flip side can't be ignored. The power to edit genes opens the door to choosing not just for health but for specific traits deemed "desirable" by society or individual parents. What happens when parents can select the height, intelligence, or even artistic abilities of their child? Beyond the ethical implications of such choices, there's the potential for a societal divide, where the rich can afford to "design" their progeny, leading to genetically enhanced elite classes, while others are left behind in the genetic lottery.

Furthermore, the science, while promising, is still in its nascent stages. Unintended consequences could emerge from genetic editing, leading to new genetic anomalies or health challenges that we haven't foreseen.

Genetic Discrimination: As our understanding of the human genome expands, so does our ability to predict an individual's likelihood of developing certain illnesses or conditions. While this knowledge could be invaluable in preventative medicine, it also introduces the peril of genetic discrimination.

For instance, employers might be reluctant to hire someone with a higher predisposition to certain diseases, fearing frequent absences or early retirement. Insurance companies could hike premiums or deny coverage altogether based on one's genetic makeup, arguing that some people are "high risk." Such scenarios could lead to a society where individuals are defined, limited, and discriminated against based on their genes rather than their abilities or character.

Furthermore, this knowledge could have psychological implications. Knowing one's predisposition might lead to a self-fulfilling prophecy where individuals limit themselves based on their genetic "destiny."

In the end, genetic engineering stands at the intersection of science and ethics. While its potential benefits are staggering, so are its pitfalls. As we forge ahead, it will be crucial to establish rigorous ethical guidelines and engage in global dialogues, ensuring that the power of genetics is harnessed for the collective good and not misused to the detriment of individual rights and societal harmony.

AI and the Sanctity of the Doctor-Patient Relationship:

As Artificial Intelligence continues to make inroads into the medical field, it brings with it a series of challenges and concerns, not just technological but deeply human. At the heart of this evolution lies the fundamental relationship between a doctor and their patient, an age-old bond built on trust, empathy, and mutual understanding. But how does this relationship fare in the age of AI?

Depersonalization of Care: The increasing reliance on AI-driven diagnostic tools and treatment recommendations has the potential to shift the dynamics of medical care. While AI systems might offer rapid and accurate diagnoses, they lack the ability to understand the nuanced emotional and psychological aspects of a patient's experience. A machine can identify a heart condition from an ECG, but it cannot sense the underlying anxieties, the personal stories, or the unique contexts in which the ailment exists. The concern, then, is whether we're heading towards a healthcare system that, while technologically advanced, misses out on the deeply human components of care. Will doctors, with their tight schedules and reliance on AI tools, lose that irreplaceable connection, the ability to comfort, empathize, and offer hope? Balancing the efficiency of AI with the irreplaceable human elements of healthcare will be paramount.

Data Privacy: AI's efficacy lies in its ability to process massive datasets to discern patterns and make predictions. Every patient interaction, every diagnostic report, every symptom becomes a data point. But as the repositories of health data grow, so does the risk of data breaches. The question then arises: Who truly owns this data? Is it the patient from whom it originates? The medical institutions that collect it? Or the tech companies that process it? The potential misuse of health data—be it for unauthorized research, targeted marketing, or even more malicious intents—becomes a pressing concern.

Beyond ownership, the sanctity and protection of this data are of utmost importance. As we integrate AI further into healthcare, robust cybersecurity measures need to be in place. We also need transparent policies and regulations to ensure that the data isn't misused and that patients retain agency over their personal health information.

Moreover, as AI systems become intermediaries in doctor-patient interactions, there's a need to ensure that these systems don't inadvertently erode the trust inherent in the relationship. Patients need to be confident that their personal stories, worries, and health data are secure and respected, even in a digitized environment.

In the evolving landscape of healthcare, AI presents both immense promise and significant challenges. While it can revolutionize how we diagnose and treat illnesses, it's crucial to remember that healthcare, at its core, is a human endeavour. Embracing the benefits of AI while upholding the sanctity of the doctor-patient relationship will be key to shaping a future that is both technologically advanced and deeply humane.

Regenerative Medicine and the Nature of Life:

Regenerative medicine, at the crossroads of biology, technology, and ethics, has the potential to redefine our understanding of life and the human experience. Its advancements promise incredible benefits but also pose philosophical, ethical, and societal questions. This exploration will delve deeper into some of the most pressing issues in the domain of regenerative medicine.

Stem Cell Research: Stem cells, with their capacity to become any type of cell in the human body, have offered a tantalizing glimpse into the potential for repairing damaged tissues and organs. Particularly, embryonic stem cells hold significant promise due to their pluripotency. However, the very nature of their origin – from embryos – has made them a focal point of ethical debates. At the heart of this discourse is the question of when life truly begins. Does an embryo, with the potential to develop into a full human, possess inherent rights and value? If so, is it justifiable to use such potential life for research, even if it may pave the way for revolutionary treatments that could save or improve countless existing lives? Ethical perspectives vary widely, from religious and moral standpoints to utilitarian views about the greater good.

Life Extension: One of the most transformative promises of regenerative medicine is its potential to significantly extend the human lifespan. While on the surface, living longer might seem like an unequivocal benefit, it raises profound questions. Firstly, should we pursue life extension simply because we can? What constitutes a life well-lived, and does stretching out the human lifespan necessarily equate to a better quality of life?

From a societal perspective, a considerably aged population presents numerous challenges. Resources, already strained in many parts of the world, could become even scarcer. Pensions, healthcare systems, and social welfare structures might become overwhelmed. Intergenerational tensions could rise, with younger generations possibly feeling the weight of an older, more dominant demographic.

Beyond the tangible, the very essence of our understanding of life and death may shift. Death, an inevitable part of the human experience, provides life with urgency, meaning, and context. If this finality were to be postponed indefinitely, how would our perceptions of accomplishments, relationships, and experiences evolve? Would an extended life lead to greater fulfillment or potentially result in existential stagnation?

In conclusion, regenerative medicine, while teeming with promise, introduces dilemmas that challenge the fabric of our moral, societal, and philosophical constructs. As we stand on the brink of potentially redefining life, it's crucial to engage in these dialogues, ensuring that the path forward is not only scientifically informed but also ethically sound and culturally sensitive.

Economic and Socio-cultural Implications:

As we venture deeper into a world shaped by advanced biomedical and technological breakthroughs, the broader implications for our economies and social fabrics become crucial areas of exploration. The exciting potential of these advancements is matched by equally compelling concerns about how they might reshape societal structures and values.

Access and Inequity: The benefits of modern science, from the most sophisticated treatments to groundbreaking procedures, carry significant costs. Such expenses run the risk of accentuating existing inequities in society. Those with the means may be able to avail themselves of treatments that could improve health, extend life, or even enhance natural abilities. The result might be an emerging class of 'enhanced' individuals with advantages not just in health, but in cognitive abilities, physical prowess, and lifespan. This poses the alarming prospect of a society bifurcating into those who can afford to 'upgrade' and those relegated to a baseline human experience. Solutions may range from policy interventions, such as subsidizing critical treatments, to innovative business models that democratize access. Yet, it remains an essential challenge to ensure that advancements benefit humanity as a whole, not just an elite few.

Changing Cultural Norms: As technology influences human capabilities and experiences, the foundational norms of societies worldwide are poised for disruption. The respect and reverence often accorded to age and accumulated wisdom might diminish in a world where age becomes a more fluid concept. If life can be significantly extended, what value does society place on youth or the traditional markers of age? Additionally, our rituals, stories, and shared experiences around the concept of life and death might be upended. A natural life trajectory, with its milestones and shared experiences, provides a framework for societal cohesion. When these milestones shift or even disappear, the challenge will be to navigate these changes without losing the shared narratives that bind communities together.

These shifts, both economic and socio-cultural, will require adaptive governance, foresight in policy-making, and an inclusive dialogue encompassing diverse stakeholders. They underline the importance of not just celebrating scientific advancements but also deeply considering the broader tapestry of societal implications they weave. As we look ahead, the pivotal task will be to harness these advancements in ways that promote collective progress and societal cohesion.

In the realm where science and wonders align,
Modern medicine whispers of times so fine.
With each step towards what the future holds dear,
In the shadows of progress, doubts begin to
appear.
Genetic codes twisted, AI by our side,
Regenerative wonders in which we confide.
Yet each marvel brings questions, profound and
deep,
Challenging beliefs that our ancestors did keep.
Designer babes rising; genes picked and refined,
The ethics of choice heavily intertwined.
The doctor and patient, once close and so clear,
Now wade through the waters of newfound
frontier.
Longevity's riddles, life's extension, and cost,
Are we playing with nature, and what could be
lost?
To balance our strides with ethics so pure,
Preserving our cultures, ensuring the cure.
This dance of progression, so vibrant, so grand,
Demands our reflection, a thoughtful hand.
With global dialogues and minds intertwined,
We'll steer this new age with humanity in mind.
For the marvels of medicine, vast and so new,
Hold promise for all, not just the select few.
Through unity and wisdom, we must chart the
seas,
To ensure that our future is one of shared peace.

CHAPTER 6:
BIOGERONTOLOGY - UNRAVELLING THE SECRETS OF AGEING

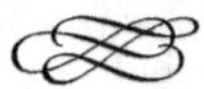

From time immemorial, ageing has been viewed as a natural, inevitable process—much like the setting of the sun at dusk. But what if the twilight years weren't as predetermined as we once thought? Enter biogerontology, the scientific arena that casts a fresh, analytical gaze upon the biology of ageing, aiming to comprehend and, perhaps, reconfigure the tapestry of our golden years.

Defining Ageing: Beyond the Chronological Clock

Ageing isn't merely about the accumulation of birthdays. Biologically, it represents a complex interplay of cellular events, genetic changes, and metabolic shifts. Some view it as a programmed sequence of events, while others see it as a result of accumulated damage. But one thing's for certain: it's far from being a mere consequence of chronological time.

The Genetics of Longevity: Inheriting the Ticks of Time

The quest for the fountain of youth may not solely rest in tales and myths; part of it might be encoded within our very DNA. Delving into the science of longevity reveals fascinating genetic tales that hint at why some individuals and species outlive their peers.

1. Family Legacies of Longevity:

Human Chronicles: Many of us have heard tales of families where multiple members live well past the age of 100. Scientific investigations validate these stories, showing that longevity tends to cluster in families, suggesting an inherited component.

Model Organisms' Tales: Scientists often turn to simpler organisms, such as the nematode *Caenorhabditis elegans*, to decipher longevity secrets. Remarkably, manipulating single genes in these organisms can double or even triple their lifespans.

2. Star Players in the Longevity Game:

FOXO: The Guardian of Longevity: The FOXO family of transcription factors regulates a wide array of processes, from glucose metabolism to cell death. In various organisms, heightened FOXO activity is associated with longer life. What's fascinating is that these genes seem to have conserved their longevity-promoting effects from worms to humans.

SIRT: The Cellular Maestros: Sirtuins, a family of proteins to which SIRT belongs, are emerging rockstars in the ageing world. They're involved in DNA repair, inflammation control, and metabolic regulation. Caloric restriction, known to extend lifespan in multiple species, seems to operate in part by activating sirtuins.

3. The Underlying Mechanisms:

DNA's Self-defense: Both FOXO and SIRT are involved in DNA repair. As organisms age, DNA damage accumulates, leading to functional decline. By enhancing repair mechanisms, these genes potentially slow down the ticking of the biological clock.

Metabolic Harmony: Ageing is closely tied to metabolism. FOXO and SIRT genes fine-tune metabolic pathways, ensuring cells extract energy efficiently and manage resources wisely, attributes often linked to extended health span.

Cellular Life and Death Decisions: Proper regulation of cell death, or apoptosis, is vital. An imbalance can result in premature ageing or cancerous growth. Longevity genes like FOXO ensure this delicate balance is maintained.

4. Bridging Genetics and Environment:

Nature vs. Nurture: While genetics provides the framework, environmental factors like diet, exercise, and stress modulate the effects of longevity genes. This interplay makes the longevity equation dynamic and multifaceted.

Gene Activation and Silencing: Certain environmental triggers can turn on or off longevity genes. For instance, diets mimicking caloric restriction can activate SIRT genes, offering a genetic boost to longevity without drastic food reduction.

By diving deep into the genetics of longevity, researchers aspire to uncover strategies to extend not just life but also the quality of it. While the dream of eternal youth remains a fantasy, understanding our genetic makeup might provide the keys to healthier, longer lives.

Cellular Senescence: The Ticking Clocks Inside Us

Deep within our bodies, on a microscopic scale, cells diligently operate to maintain the equilibrium of life. Yet, like intricate timepieces, their mechanisms are susceptible to wear and tear. As the ticks of these cellular clocks wind down, we face the phenomenon of senescence.

1. Understanding Cellular Timekeeping:

Natural Lifecycle: Just as every living organism has a lifecycle, so too do cells. They grow, divide, and sometimes retire into a state of senescence. While this process is natural, it becomes problematic when senescent cells accumulate.

Hallmarks of Senescence: Senescent cells exhibit distinctive characteristics—they enlarge, their internal structures rearrange, and they release certain chemicals into their surroundings.

2. Consequences of Accumulated Senescence:

Toxic Neighbors: Although they are inert in terms of growth, senescent cells are not silent bystanders. They release inflammatory and damaging compounds, termed senescence-associated secretory phenotype (SASP), which can negatively impact neighboring healthy cells.

Tissue Breakdown: As more cells enter senescence, tissue repair and regeneration decline. This can lead to the thinning of skin, weakening of bones, and other age-related ailments.

3. The Silver Lining: Evolutionary Perspective:

Short-term Benefits: Ironically, senescence evolved as a protective mechanism. By preventing damaged cells from dividing, it reduces the risk of cancerous growth.

Long-term Trade-offs: However, while beneficial in youth, the accumulation of senescent cells over a lifetime might tip the balance towards ageing and disease.

4. Reversing the Cellular Clock: The Promise of Research:

Clearing Out the Old: Scientists are exploring drugs termed senolytics, which selectively eliminate senescent cells. Early studies in mice show that clearing these cells can reverse signs of ageing and extend the health span.

Rejuvenation: Instead of just removing senescent cells, some research focuses on rejuvenating them, restoring their normal function, and effectively turning back their internal clocks.

5. Implications for Age-related Diseases:

Inflammation and Disease: Many age-related diseases, from arthritis to Alzheimer's, have links to inflammation. With senescent cells being a source of chronic inflammation, tackling them might offer therapeutic avenues.

Tissue Regeneration: By managing cellular senescence, we might also enhance the body's ability to repair and regenerate, paving the way for treatments that not only extend lifespan but also ensure vitality in later years.

The exploration into cellular senescence provides a deeper understanding of the very fabric of ageing. As we learn more about these internal timekeepers, the possibility emerges: can we truly recalibrate the clocks within our cells?

Metabolic Pathways: Powering the Journey Through Time

The delicate dance of metabolic processes within our cells serves as the backbone of our vitality. It's a harmonious ballet of energy production and usage, responding keenly to external factors like diet and, in turn, influencing our rate of ageing. Pivotal pathways, like mTOR and AMPK, become the conductors of this metabolic orchestra, with the potential to shape our journey through time.

1. Metabolic Processes: A Brief Overview

Dietary Influence: Every morsel of food we consume is broken down and channeled into various metabolic pathways, which are essentially the cell's machinery for generating and using energy.

Cellular Energetics: Beyond just energy, these pathways dictate cellular health, determining the balance between growth, repair, and recycling.

2. The Role of mTOR: The Growth Conductor

Nutrient Detection: mTOR (Mechanistic Target of Rapamycin) acts like a vigilant sentinel, detecting nutrient abundance, particularly amino acids, and insulin signals.

Driving Growth: When nutrients are plentiful, mTOR promotes cell growth and protein synthesis but dials down autophagy—a cellular "clean-up" process.

Implications for Ageing: Continuous activation of mTOR due to excessive nutrient intake might accelerate ageing by reducing the cell's focus on repair and maintenance.

3. AMPK: The Guardian of Energy Scarcity

Sensing Energy Shortage: AMPK (AMP-activated protein kinase) springs into action when the cell's energy (often detected as low ATP levels) is running low.

Promotion of Autophagy: As a counterpoint to mTOR, AMPK promotes autophagy, ensuring that cells recycle damaged components and generate energy.

Protective Role in Ageing: By boosting cellular maintenance and energy production, AMPK activation might help counteract some of the detrimental effects of ageing.

4. Manipulating the Metabolic Maestros for Longevity

Dietary Interventions: Caloric restriction, or reducing food intake without malnutrition, has been shown to decrease mTOR activity while boosting AMPK. This dietary strategy has extended lifespans in numerous organisms, from yeast to mammals.

Pharmacological Avenues: Drugs like rapamycin (targeting mTOR) and metformin (linked to AMPK activation) are being studied for their potential to mimic the lifespan-extending effects of caloric restriction.

5. The Balance of Metabolism and Ageing

Fine-tuning the System: Ageing can be viewed as an outcome of the equilibrium between growth and maintenance, influenced by our metabolic processes.

Future Promise: As we uncover more about these pathways, personalized interventions might be developed to optimize our metabolic balance and potentially delay the ageing process.

In essence, our metabolic pathways are not just about powering our daily activities; they're intricately woven into the tapestry of our ageing journey. Through understanding and potentially adjusting these internal mechanisms, we might find avenues to travel through time with grace and vitality.

The Potential of Interventions: Navigating Uncharted Seas

In the quest for longevity, we have unearthed a trove of compounds and molecules that show potential in stalling or even reversing the ageing tide. Metformin, traditionally used to combat diabetes, has emerged as a frontrunner in this arena, with studies suggesting its prowess in extending lifespan. Rapamycin, another molecule, has shown promise in regulating ageing's critical pathways, further expanding our anti-ageing arsenal.

1. The Allure of Metformin: Beyond Diabetes

Mode of Action: Metformin's anti-ageing effects stem from its ability to activate the AMPK pathway, promoting cellular repair and energy balance.

Benefits Observed: Studies in organisms ranging from worms to mammals have shown an extension in lifespan and healthspan with metformin usage.

Implications for Humans: Preliminary research suggests metformin could decrease the incidence of age-related diseases in humans, potentially offering more years of healthy life.

2. Rapamycin: The Gatekeeper of Youth?

Unveiling its Secrets: Originally discovered in the soils of Easter Island, rapamycin's primary role was as an immunosuppressant. Its impact on the mTOR pathway, however, catapulted it into the spotlight of anti-ageing research.

Impacting Ageing Pathways: By inhibiting the mTOR pathway, rapamycin can tilt the balance in favour of cellular repair and autophagy, potentially slowing ageing.

Studies and Results: Research in mice has shown that rapamycin can extend lifespan, paving the way for human trials.

3. Navigating the Waters with Caution

Understanding Side Effects: While these interventions harbour promise, they come with their baggage. For instance, rapamycin, being an immunosuppressant, might increase susceptibility to infections.

Long-term Implications: The long-term effects of such interventions, especially in humans, are still a grey area. Continuous research and monitoring are vital to ensure they don't introduce new age-related complications.

Personalized Approaches: The efficacy and safety of these interventions could vary based on genetics, lifestyle, and existing health conditions. As research progresses, tailoring treatments to individuals might become essential.

In the vast ocean of anti-ageing research, these interventions represent exciting new vessels. But like any voyage into unknown waters, it's vital to navigate with both hope and prudence, ensuring we don't sacrifice safety in our pursuit of extended youth.

Striking the Balance: Longevity and Life's Worth

While the allure of a longer life captivates many, the quality of those extended years takes precedence. It's not about simply stretching out time, but enriching the tapestry of experiences within it. Interventions in the realm of longevity should be evaluated not just by the years they add, but by the life they breathe into those years.

1. **Defining Healthspan:** It goes beyond mere survival. Healthspan encompasses the years an individual lives without debilitating diseases, enjoying mental clarity, physical vitality, and emotional well-being. It's about savouring life's moments, unburdened by ailments that often accompany ageing.

2. **The Promise and Peril of Interventions:** While drugs like metformin and rapamycin show potential in extending life, their true value lies in their capacity to prolong the healthspan. Any intervention's merits should be weighed against its risks—

does it merely add years, or does it enhance the quality of those years?

3. **Holistic Well-being:** Physical health is just one facet of a fulfilling life. Cognitive function, emotional balance, and social connections also play pivotal roles. Interventions should be seen as part of a broader strategy, complemented by mental exercises, social engagement, and emotional well-being practices.

4. **Ethical Considerations:** Prolonging life also brings with it ethical dilemmas. As we push the boundaries of human lifespan, questions about resource allocation, societal roles, and inter-generational equity arise. It's crucial to navigate these waters with foresight and empathy.

In the quest for longevity, it's paramount to ensure that life remains vibrant, meaningful, and worth living. The dance of life isn't just about the number of steps, but the passion and joy with which they're taken.

Navigating the Waters of Extended Lifespans: Societal and Ethical Reverberations

As science propels us closer to the reality of significantly extended lifespans, we are urged to reevaluate the constructs of our society and confront complex ethical dilemmas.

1. **Rethinking Retirement and Economic Systems:** Traditional retirement ages were set with average lifespans in mind. If people live longer, healthier lives, will they work longer? How would this impact job opportunities for younger generations? Our pension systems, predicated on specific age benchmarks, would need drastic recalibration to ensure sustainability.

2. **Intergenerational Dynamics:** Longer lifespans mean more generations coexisting simultaneously. This could enrich our societies with diverse perspectives but also potentially lead to conflicts. Issues like housing, resource allocation, and political power dynamics might tilt as older generations retain their influence longer.

3. **Environmental and Resource Implications:** Our planet's resources are already under strain. If lifespans significantly increase, the demand for resources, from food to housing, would escalate, potentially exacerbating issues like climate change, unless sustainable solutions are simultaneously pursued.

4. **Societal Stratification and Access:** Will life-extending interventions be accessible to everyone or become the privilege of the affluent? There's a

risk of widening societal disparities if only a segment of the population can afford these treatments, leading to a bifurcated society: those who live longer and those who don't.

5. **The Value of Life:** Philosophically, an extended life beckons the question of life's intrinsic value. Does a longer life equate to a more meaningful one? Or could it dilute the significance of our experiences, milestones, and relationships?

6. **The Moral Quandary:** At the heart of these advancements lies a profound ethical question: just because we can extend life, does it mean we should? And who gets to decide the answer?

These considerations implore us to approach the prospects of extended life holistically. It's not just a scientific endeavour but an intricate weave of societal, philosophical, and ethical threads. As we look to the horizon of potential human evolution, it's paramount to tread thoughtfully, balancing the allure of scientific advancements with the depth of their implications.

In the vast domain where life's secrets reside,
Biogerontology stands, with eyes open wide.
More than science, it's a journey profound,
Into humanity's core, where truths are unbound.

Before us lies a vision, so tempting and bright,
Of extended days and health shining light.
Yet, with such power, comes a duty so grand,
To wield it with care, with a steady hand.

Navigating waters, where no charts have been
drawn,
In search of longevity's promising dawn.
Our compass must twirl, true and unfazed,
By knowledge, ethics, and passion ablaze.

Seeking not just years, but life of great worth,
Filled with depth, purpose, and vibrant rebirth.
So as we journey, let's vow to embrace,
Every challenge and joy in this wondrous race.

CHAPTER 7: THE TAO OF AGEING: ANCIENT WISDOM IN MODERN TIMES

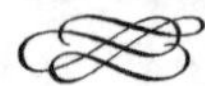

In the bustling progress of biomedicine, it's easy to become enamoured with the marvels of technology and science. However, as we look to reshape the contours of human ageing, it's worth revisiting ancient philosophies that have contemplated the nature of life, ageing, and balance for millennia. Among these, the Tao, or Dao, rooted in Chinese philosophy and central to Taoism, offers profound insights that can enrich our understanding of the ageing process.

The Tao: Embracing Nature's Rhythms and Life's Transitions

Central to Taoist thought is the concept of Tao, often translated as 'the way' or 'path'. It's more than just a direction or a route; it encapsulates the ineffable, intrinsic essence and rhythm of the universe. Rooted in the ancient wisdom of Chinese philosophy, Tao beckons one to align with the universe's natural currents, to navigate life with ease and grace, much like water flows seamlessly around obstacles, seeking its own level.

The philosophy accentuates the importance of living in sync with nature's cadence. It advises not to resist or defy the natural order but to adapt, adjust, and assimilate, finding serenity in the cosmic dance of creation, sustenance, and dissolution.

When viewed through the prism of ageing, Taoism offers a profound perspective. Ageing, in the Taoist worldview, is not an anomaly or a challenge to be conquered. Instead, it is an integral chapter of the grand narrative of life—a chapter replete with its own set of experiences, teachings, and wisdom. Just as the seasons seamlessly transition from spring's vitality to winter's dormancy, our lives too ebb and flow, with ageing being an inevitable tide in this continuum.

Fighting this natural process or viewing it solely as an adversary is a futile endeavor, akin to attempting to halt the flow of a mighty river. Instead, Taoism encourages a reframe: to view ageing as an ally, a phase of introspection, maturity, and deeper understanding. It's a time to reap the harvest of years gone by, to cherish memories, to embrace the silver linings, and to impart wisdom to younger generations.

In essence, aligning with the Tao in the context of ageing means recognizing and celebrating this phase as a natural, enriching, and inherent facet of existence. It nudges us to approach ageing not with apprehension, but with acceptance and grace, finding beauty in every wrinkle, story in every scar, and wisdom in every gray hair.

Yin and Yang: Navigating the Harmonious Dance of Polarities

At the epicenter of Taoist thought lies the enigmatic but essential interplay between Yin and Yang. These two forces, though appearing to be polar opposites, intertwine in a complex ballet, illustrating the interconnected and interdependent nature of life's multifaceted tapestry. They are not isolated entities but parts of a greater whole, each one constantly shaping and being shaped by the other, echoing the cyclical and symbiotic patterns found throughout the universe.

Aging, when seen through this Taoist lens, becomes a symphony of contrasts. The exuberant energy and forward momentum of Yang symbolize the phases of growth, exploration, and expansion in one's life journey. It represents the moments of seizing opportunities, the exhilarating peaks of accomplishments, and the audacity to break boundaries and challenge norms.

In contrast, Yin encapsulates the often understated, tranquil elegance of decline. It isn't merely about physical slowing down but also encompasses the deep introspection, the cherishing of memories, and the gentle acceptance of life's impermanence. Yin, with its introspective quality, calls upon the individual to look inward, to savor the accumulated wisdom of the years, and to find contentment and peace in the ebb and flow of existence.

Yet, in our modern epoch, there's a palpable tilt towards glorifying the Yang aspects of life. Modern medicine, with its technological prowess, frequently focuses on prolonging life's timeline, frequently at the risk of diminishing its depth. There's an overarching ambition to push the boundaries of human longevity, often sidelining the profound experiences and insights that accompany the Yin phase of aging.

To truly appreciate the entirety of the human experience, we must learn to navigate and harmonize with both these forces. Recognizing the inherent value in each phase — the vibrancy of Yang and the depth of Yin — is imperative. By doing so, not only can medical endeavors be enhanced, embracing a more holistic approach to well-being, but society at large can gain a renewed appreciation for life's complete journey. This richer understanding challenges us to perceive aging not as a one-dimensional decline but as a layered, enriching process, offering insights into the very core of existence and what it means to be fully alive.

Wu Wei: Embracing Effortless Action and Nature's Dance

Deeply entrenched in Taoist thought, Wu Wei stands as a testament to the philosophy of effortless action — a seemingly paradoxical concept that marries purposeful intention with the grace of letting go. Transcending mere idleness or inaction, Wu Wei captures the nuanced art of moving in alignment with the universe's inherent patterns and rhythms. It's about understanding the delicate balance between pushing and yielding, between acting and refraining.

Imagine a tree, steadfast and resilient, yet bending and swaying in response to the winds, never fighting against them but adapting harmoniously. Such is the spirit of Wu Wei: to engage with life not as a battle to be won, but as a dance to be enjoyed, feeling out the tempo and joining in its rhythm.

In the context of ageing, this philosophy takes on a particularly profound resonance. The process of growing older, with its myriad challenges and transformations, becomes a canvas upon which the principles of Wu Wei can be vividly painted. It promotes a mindful understanding of ageing: to view it not as a relentless foe, but as a natural counterpart to growth and evolution.

Wu Wei instills in us the wisdom to differentiate between moments that necessitate proactive intervention and those where passive observation or acceptance serves best. For instance, while medical interventions may sometimes be necessary to address health concerns in ageing, there are also times when one's well-being is best served by simply accepting and embracing the natural processes of the body and mind. It's about knowing when to actively steer the course of our life and when to let the currents take us where they will.

As we age, Wu Wei becomes an essential compass, guiding us to find equilibrium. This philosophy fosters a balanced perspective on ageing — one where we aren't merely passive observers of time's passage but active participants in a journey that we navigate with grace, understanding, and ease. Through Wu Wei, we learn that sometimes the most potent action is found in the gentle embrace of life's natural flow.

The Tao's Embrace of Simplicity and Contentment: Crafting A Legacy of Fulfillment

In the vast tapestry of Eastern thought, the Tao emerges as a beacon, illuminating the path towards a life characterized by simplicity, harmony, and profound contentment. This ancient wisdom, while timeless in its essence, finds particular relevance in the twilight years of human existence, as individuals navigate the nuanced terrains of age, introspection, and legacy.

As the sun begins its descent on the horizon of our lives, the Tao's teachings beckon us to embrace a recalibrated approach to living. The inexorable march of time, with its ever-shifting landscapes, offers a poignant reminder of the impermanent nature of all things. In this phase, the act of decluttering morphs from a mere practice into a transformative philosophy. It's not just about discarding the tangible — the excess possessions that clutter our living spaces — but also about unburdening the intangible weights that have perhaps anchored our spirits: unresolved resentments, unmet expectations, and unfulfilled aspirations.

Choosing simplicity, as championed by the Tao, becomes an exercise in discernment and intentionality. It's about recognizing that in the vast sea of life's possibilities, not everything that glitters holds value. Embracing minimalism in this context is far from a life of deprivation; it's a journey towards essence. It's a conscious curation of life, a decision to surround oneself with not just what's good, but what's truly meaningful.

Contentment, a virtue often misunderstood as complacency, is in the Taoist perspective a celebration of the present. It's an acknowledgment and appreciation of the here and now, irrespective of its imperfections. By cultivating contentment amidst simplicity, individuals open the doors to a realm where every moment is savored, where joys are magnified, and where the tapestry of life, woven with threads of experiences, is viewed in its holistic beauty.

As we approach the golden chapters of our existence, these Taoist ideals stand as invaluable guides, nudging us towards a sanctuary of peace and enrichment. They serve as reminders that in the ebbing tides of life, amidst its complexities and uncertainties, lies an opportunity: to live with purpose, to cherish with gratitude, and to age with grace.

The Tao of Medicine: Embracing Equilibrium in Healing

Modern medicine, with its vast arsenal of techniques and technologies, has often portrayed ailments and the inescapable journey of ageing as adversaries in a relentless battle, where victory is equated with dominance, suppression, and control. While undeniably effective in many instances, this approach occasionally risks reducing the patient to a mere battleground of symptoms, potentially sidelining their holistic well-being.

Enter the Taoist perspective — a gentle reminder of the age-old wisdom rooted in harmony, balance, and the interconnectivity of all things. Taoism, rather than placing us at odds with our health challenges, invites us to engage with them in a dance of understanding and alignment. This philosophy doesn't propagate passive surrender or a defeatist attitude towards diseases or ageing. Instead, it carves out a path that recognizes and honors the interconnected web of physical, emotional, mental, and spiritual dimensions that constitute human existence.

From the Taoist lens, interventions in health are not about launching aggressive offensives against perceived threats. They pivot towards a more nuanced and compassionate approach. The focus shifts from mere symptom alleviation to understanding the root causes, from silencing the discord to harmonizing the melody of one's being. It's akin to tuning a musical instrument — not by force, but by attentive and gentle adjustments, ensuring each note resonates in its purest form.

Embracing the Tao in medicine challenges the healthcare paradigm to expand its horizons. It nudges practitioners and patients alike to view health as more than just the absence of disease. It's about fostering an environment where the body and mind can naturally recalibrate, restoring their intrinsic balance. This approach doesn't dismiss the value of modern medical interventions but supplements them with a philosophy that prioritizes nurturing over combating, equilibrium over extremes.

In essence, the Tao of Medicine is a clarion call for a medical ethos where the journey to healing is as revered as the destination, where the symphony of human experience is valued as much as the final outcome. It's a vision of healthcare where patients are not just bodies to be treated but souls to be understood, and where healing is a collaborative dance of harmony and grace.

Taoism and the Quest for Immortality: The Eternal Essence Beyond Temporality

In the vast expanse of scientific exploration, biogerontology emerges as a discipline deeply engrossed in decoding the mysteries of ageing. It seeks answers in the microscopic dance of cells, genes, and proteins, aiming to extend the ticking clock of our biological existence. Often, this scientific pilgrimage centers on the pursuit of adding more candles to our birthday cakes, accentuating the quantitative aspects of life's journey.

Taoism, on the other hand, introduces a transformative perspective on immortality, one that challenges our conventional interpretations. Instead of viewing immortality as a ceaseless extension of physical existence, it redirects our gaze towards realms more profound and ethereal. In Taoist thought, immortality isn't necessarily about the incessant beating of the heart, but about the heart's unbroken connection to the cosmic rhythm of the Tao.

This unique conception of immortality is less about persisting in time and more about transcending it. It's about attaining a state of spiritual enlightenment wherein the individual soul commingles with the vastness of the universe, experiencing a deep resonance and oneness with the Tao. In this harmonious fusion, distinctions between the self and the cosmos blur, and one finds eternity not in years or decades but in the timeless embrace of the universe.

The Taoist pursuit of immortality underscores the idea that life's true essence isn't encapsulated in its duration but in its depth. It's about imbibing the richness of experiences, the profundity of insights, and the interconnectedness of all existence. It's not about how many sunrises one witnesses, but about the quality of stillness and reflection one finds in each dawn. In this philosophical framework, every fleeting moment holds the potential for infinity.

In sum, Taoism's perspective on immortality serves as a profound reminder: It invites us to search for eternity not in the endless corridors of time but in the boundless depths of each moment. It encourages us to seek not just longevity but a life imbued with meaning, essence, and connection. In the dance of existence, it's not the number of steps that matter, but the soul with which each step is taken.

Immortality, in this light, is about being eternally present, cherishing the infinite within the finite.

In the eons of existence, our temporal lives are but
fleeting sparks,
Yet within each moment, the Tao's wisdom
embarks.
Ageing, not as an end but a transition to embrace,
Guided by ancient teachings, we find our place.

The balance of Yin and Yang, a dance so profound,
In the rhythms of life, their harmonies are found.
In the Yin of introspection and the Yang of our
might,
Ageing emerges in a new, radiant light.

Wu Wei's teachings, so effortlessly true,
Remind us to flow, to yield, to pursue.
With acceptance and grace, through every life
stage,
We find harmony, wisdom, and sage.

Medicine's quest, to heal and to mend,
Finds depth in the Tao, a timeless friend.
In this union, a path unfolds,
Where healing is a story beautifully told.

Immortality, a concept so vast and so deep,
Is redefined by the Tao, a secret we keep.
Not in years or decades, but in moments so fine,
We find eternity, in every heartbeat's line.

In the dance of existence, in the vast cosmic sea,

The Tao teaches us to be, to see.
In the heartbeats, in whispers, in silent reprieve,
Ageing, through the Tao, is a tapestry we weave.

Let us cherish each step, each memory, each tear,
For in the Tao's embrace, there's nothing to fear.
With grace, with wisdom, with timeless delight,
We journey forward, bathed in the Tao's gentle
light.

CONCLUSION

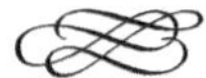

A Vision for an Ethical Medical Future

As we stand at the precipice of a new era in medicine, one imbued with remarkable technological advancements and transformative treatments; it's clear that our journey is as much about introspection as it is about innovation. The chapters of this exposé, spanning from the cutting-edge vistas of regenerative medicine and artificial intelligence to the timeless wisdom of the Tao, have elucidated both the monumental promises of modern medicine and the profound ethical challenges accompanying them.

Humanity's quest has always been about pushing boundaries, seeking longer, healthier, and more fulfilled lives. With each stride in biogerontology and each algorithm of AI, the age-old adage resonates even more: "Just because we can, doesn't always mean we should." The paradigms we establish

now are not just for our immediate era but will
guide generations to come.

A few guiding principles emerge from our exploration:

1. **The Balance of Intervention and Acceptance:** As science offers transformative treatments, ancient philosophies like the Tao underscore the significance of acceptance and graceful ageing.

2. **Inclusive Dialogue:** Today's decisions require collective wisdom. Ethicists, medical professionals, patients, technologists, policymakers, and the public must collaboratively shape the medical landscape.

3. **Ensuring Equity:** Advancements in medicine should not become tools of division. Every individual, irrespective of their socioeconomic status, deserves access to the best care.

4. **Education and Awareness:** Demystifying complex treatments for the general populace ensures informed decision-making and trust in medical progress.

5. **Preserving Humanity:** While we harness AI and technological marvels, healthcare's essence remains human. Empathy, understanding, and compassion should always be at the heart of care.

6. **Continuous Ethical Review**: With the rapid pace of medical and technological evolution, dynamic ethical guidelines are paramount. Regular reviews will be essential to address emerging challenges.

In weaving together the tapestry of this exposé, from the intricacies of cellular regeneration to the wisdom of ancient philosophies, we are imbued with a sentiment of awe and responsibility. The horizon of possibilities is vast, but our best compass remains the ageless ethos of 'do no harm.' It's the synthesis of innovation with a deep respect for life that will ensure a future where medicine serves not just the individual but the very soul of humanity.

In the whisper of the Tao, nature speaks,
Beyond mountains high and valleys deep.
The rhythm of life, a dance so profound,
Where boundaries blur, and spirits unbound.

With every breath, the Yin and the Yang,
Balance life's journey, with a silent clang.
Yet man aspires, with eyes cast above,
To break free from chains, to soar like a dove.

But within the Tao, wisdom does lie,
That to truly transcend, one must comply,
With the ebb and the flow, the moon and the tide,
For in nature's embrace, true strength resides.

Though our flesh may age, and our steps grow
slow,
The spirit remains with an eternal glow.
By embracing the Tao and nature's decree,
We transcend our limits, becoming truly free.

www.ingramcontent.com/pod-product-compliance
Lightning Source LLC
Chambersburg PA
CBHW071547150726
48000CB00002B/966